MY EPILEPSY
ANGEL

Genelle Manso

DEDICATION

I would like to give a special thank you to a good dear friend and fellow author Marc Hoberman. We grew up in the same county, Rockland county New York to be exact. He has no idea how much strength he has given Isaiah and myself after reading his book that might I add he personally autographed to my son. His book search and seizure has given us both so much more into faith and growth.

I want Marc to know we will forever be grateful to him for sharing his testimony and story with not just us but with the world.

I also want to thank my Facebook group Epilepsy angels. I love you all and I'm here to tell you we started out as friends but we are now family.

To my sister Tia Benjamin, I love you sissy now and forever. Mommy Rosemary Benjamin thank you for your patience and love you give to me. And to my sister Kandy Benjamin RIP- December, 27th 2015 I love and miss you dearly. I know you are an heaven.

.

INTRODUCTION

Sometimes life throws you a curve ball or two but it is up to you to decide Either to pick the ball up and move forward or leave the ball down and just give up.

For a while there I thought my son was just stop and give up. But with the help of

myself and his dad, life for Isaiah. Epilepsy is not an easy condition to live with. I

see it first hand with Isaiah struggling every day. The uncertainties of not knowing an Absence seizure or grand mal will come on is very nerve racking.

Over the years I have learned from my dear friend Author Marc Hoberman of Search and seizure that giving up is not an option. Giving up is not an option. And here's my final thought. I tell Isaiah everyday "You have epilepsy, epilepsy doesn't have you."

ACKNOWLEDGMENTS

Thank you, Kevin Edwards, for giving me such an amazing son. We truly have a gift from God who has shown us both the true meaning of courage and bravery

1 CHAPTER

I can remember the accident like it was yesterday, it all happened so fast. I still see flashbacks to that cold day of Sunday, December 20, 2009. It was about minus 12 that day and it was freezing. My husband had decided to turn on the wood-burning stove which is like one of the best sources of heat living in the Poconos and also the cheapest. We had called the heating company that day to deliver some propane but they were backed up from all the calls they had received and let us know that they wouldn't be able to get to us until the next day. I was thankful for the stove we had, all you had to do was load some wood into it and strike a match. The wood stove was lit and it felt so nice and toasty in the house upstairs as well as downstairs and we all were doing our own thing in the house. My son and Kevin my husband was cooking breakfast and watching television and my daughter and I were upstairs in my room talking girl talk and picking out an outfit for me to wear because I had a company party to go too later that night. And that's when this is the day that changed my life and his life as well for the better and forever. Sunday afternoon I was upstairs talking to my daughter and getting ready to pick out something to wear to my company party later on that day when I hear my ex-husband scream out to me "-Genelle" not realizing it was as serious as it was I continued talking to my daughter until I hear complete silence. My ex and I weren't on the best of terms at all. We hardly talked to one another, and I had so much anger and hurt towards him that when he did talk to me I really wasn't present nor listening for that matter. We were cordial for the kids' sake and tried to not argue or raise our voices but although it became so hard for me sometimes, I did it, for my kids. I decide to finally run downstairs to see what he was calling me about and there he held my son Isaiah in his arms, his body so lifeless and still. I screamed out" What did you do?" I look back at what I asked him now and I feel bad for asking it because I know he would never do anything to our children to hurt them but it was just the first thing that came out of my mouth. When I tell people the story I almost feel it necessary to explain why I asked him that. Some people tell me it's just a natural reaction and sometimes we say things out of surprise that we would not normally say or ask. If I didn't say it to you before I am saying it now. "I'm sorry". When I looked at my son I saw nothing but bone. The color of his skin complexion is a dark brown caramel color and when I saw his face and all I could see was white. As I looked at his face all I could see was his face and the skin from his whole left side was all off and it was white. At that time, I hadn't seen his hand and I could do was scream. Screaming and crying and looking over at his dad all I can remember is him standing there very still like, as if he was in a trans. I'm yelling at him "Kevin ", "Kevin" Help me, help him" Do something" and as I kept screaming and yelling, he just stood there. Now I know he was in pure shock because one moment he's talking to Isaiah and the next minute everything changed. My son had a seizure and had fallen on our wood burning stove and got third degree burns to his face and hand. At the time we didn't realize that is what took place because that was the first seizure we have ever see him have. I called 911 and they asked me" what's your address?" and I cried "I don't know" I couldn't think I was frozen. "Is he breathing they asked?" "Yes, I replied". I guess they traced the call because they were there really fast and asking us questions but we didn't know what happened. My ex-husband was talking to the Emergency response team and he explained that had his face turned away from him and that they were talking while Isaiah was watching television and eating his breakfast which was chicken nuggets his favorite food at the time. My son didn't answer him when he asked him a question so he turned around to see why and he saw him stuck to the wood burning stove. As he continued to tell them what happened I could see the fear and the hurt on his face and he was just sobbing as he told the story. I on the other hand just kept screaming and running around the house trying to put clothes on so I could go to the hospital with my son in the ambulance. My daughter Destiny was crying and screaming as well, seeing her little brother like that just tore her up inside and as we both ran away the house they began to wheel my son out the house onto the stretcher and they were rushing him. All I could think about was what happened and if my son was going to die. I have never seen anything like that and as a mother my heart hurt to see my child going through what he had just been through.

We made it to the hospital in less than twenty minutes but to me it felt like eternity and while I was in the back of the ambulance with Isaiah and says to me "Mommy I will be okay, really please don't be upset" At that moment I knew I had to hold it together for my kid so I held in my cry and took the tissues I had in my sweatpants from I don't know when and wiped my tears from my eyes. I knew I had a strong kid but this was just too much, too much for anyone to be going through. Too much for a kid that is good, that doesn't get into any trouble, and that many people adore. As I sat in the back with him I remember thinking to myself Why him God, why him?

We arrived at the hospital and they took him right away. We had a male nurse and to my memory he wasn't very friendly. After several hours of being there and giving him heavy medication, we were told that he was being transferred to a hospital that specialized in burns. They could not help my son. Just when we were being told that, his nurse I call him nurse cachet asked if he could talk to my ex-husband and me alone. We agreed and we followed him into a small room with chairs and a table and he closed the door. He begins to ask us questions again like the ems did. "Can you tell me what happened? He has asked, we don't know what happened we already explained this, we both said at the same time. "Well he says and as he talks to us he has this little attitude, almost like a bitchy woman attitude and continues on to say" well I have to call child protective services and write a report. "Its standard procedure he says with a smirk look on his face as if he didn't believe what we told him and about ten other people. Okay I said, that's fine, we are foster parents and they all know and love us and when they see the report they will know something had to happen. I snatched his little report that he was handing me to sign and crumbled it up and put it in my pocket." The nerve of him I said to Kevin." He's a pure ass. He just shook his head as he agreed with me and we returned to my son and waited for the new ambulance to take us to the new hospital where Isaiah would be getting treated.

Finally, a doctor they called that specialized in burns came to see Isaiah and asked us what happened and we began to tell her the story like we had to the rest of the hundredth people we already told and that's when she explained that this sounded like it had a seizure." A seizure I yelled?" Yes, she said does he have any history of seizures? Uh no. "oh wait yes he did have one last week at school I said". I started telling about how he school called me at work in the morning and I can remember the call so vivid because when the nurse called me the first thing she said was "Mrs. Edwards?" Yes, this is she I said with eagerness to know what the call was about. "I have Isaiah in my office," and then there was a very awkward pause and I could hear the upset in her voice. This is she I said louder, I started to get annoyed not so much at her but I knew something was wrong and I wanted to know already. "Isaiah had a seizure about ten minutes ago in his art class "excuse me I interrupted her and said "You sure its Isaiah you have? Because Isaiah doesn't have seizures" Yes its him and yes he had a seizure she said" I actually watched him "Then she began to tell me how he was in class and the teacher went to ask him a question and he had this stare so he approached Isaiah closer and realized that he wasn't present and just as he went to touch him Isaiah fell to the ground and he instructed one of the kids in the class to run and get the nurse. She then proceeded to tell me that when she got to the class he was on the floor, his eyes were rolling, his body shaking and he was foaming at the mouth. She told me how she counted how long it was from the time she reached the class and that it was two minutes long and after it was over she put him on his side." Okay I said: I will be there right now and take him to the hospital. Okay she said and she let me know that he seemed fine now. After the seizure was over she asked him some questions like what was his name, and did he know who she was and where he was at? He knew all of the above. I hung up the phone and my heart felt like it was going to jump out my chest, my hands were shaking as I hung up the phone and my body felt like it was going to collapse. I walked away from my desk and went straight to my boss's office and explained to her what the school nurse had just explained to me. She told me to go punch out and go and to make sure I let her know what happens. That was one thing I was blessed about. Having a great boss. She didn't have kids I don't think but when it came to family, she always made us as employees feel comfortable if we had a problem and let us go handle it. If you are reading this Ms. Pamela, thank you for being patient with me, I do appreciate everything you did for me. I punched out and I ran to my car and it felt like it was taking me forever to get to the school. From my job to the elementary school it takes fifteen minutes but for some reason it seemed like it took forever. I finally reached the school and signed in and told the door monitor that I was there to pick my son up from the nurse. She handed me a parent pass and in less than ten seconds I was in the office. There my baby was laying on the nurse's cot and as soon as I opened door I ran to him. "Are you okay? "Yes, mom I'm okay". "Well what happened I asked him" "I don't know he said, I was in art class and they said I had a seizure he couldn't say the name so I helped him "seizure?" Yeah that he said seizure but I didn't he said. and I went and picked him up but first I talked with the school nurse and she said she was with him after he had one so I took him straight to the emergency hospital the same one where the nurse reported my ex-husband and I to child welfare. And after hours of tests they found nothing and sent us home. But I kept him home for a week from school to watch him doctor I said and he had nothing that I saw. Then this happens. Well she says this is what it sounds like happened how and we will take further testing. But now for the bad news she says and I could see in her eyes the pain she felt for us as well as for Isaiah. The burns he has he will always have, he's going to need surgery, she continues to explain that the burns were third degree to the bone and the reason he's not in that much pain is because it's to the bone there's no tissue or feeling left.

My son spent months in the burn center in Lehigh valley hospital in Allentown PA for treatment and had many surgeries for his face and hand. He used to tell me" well mom I think God did this for a reason", doesn't cry he would say. At age 11 he was like a little man which we still call him at age 19 now. God doesn't give us anything we can't handle, there's a purpose for me he would say. After the long hospital stay we know had to get treated for his seizures which took different medications to treat and many heartaches in between because it seemed like we were in the Doctor's Office all the time. His face looks fantastic, the skin grafts the doctor gave did for him was simply amazing and people can be cruel but Isaiah when asked what happened gives them either what he calls the five-cent story, which is the short version of what happened, or the five-dollar story which is everything that happened. He has such patients with people although he is such a quiet to himself kind of kid. I admire him for that.

My son is my hero being able to go through all of this and still does and he wants to help other children going through what he has to daily. He wants to write a book and tell his story, he wants to start a foundation for epilepsy to raise more awareness and wants to meet Bobby flay one day his idol. He wants to own a restaurant one day. This kid is amazing and will always be my hero

2 CHAPTER

The accident really messed with Isaiah's mind, which I totally understand. But for me it messed with not only my mind but it hurt my heart too. Everything I see that resembles wood stoves or fireplaces brings flashbacks and gives me bad dreams at night. I know I need therapy and I've been considering going more and more as the years go by. I have developed anxiety and one day I had what I thought was a heart attack which turned out to be an anxiety attack. I was at home and from what I can recall from the events that day where I felt dizzy, I had a great pain in my chest, I felt like I was going to pass out. My daughter Destiny had to drive me to the hospital which at that time was called Pocono Medical center now recently called Lehigh Valley hospital-Pocono. I checked in and I was called right away into a room where I put on the lovely gown, you know the one where you have to put on backwards and your backside sticks out. Isaiah kept telling "mommy it will be okay". I smiled but I was scared as hell. In my

mind I was thinking who's going to take care of me children?
Destiny I knew would be okay she was very mature for her age but
Isaiah had epilepsy.

Who's going to make all of his appointments, fill all of his
prescriptions and watch him as he slept.

The Doctor comes in and ask all the usual questions they ask you
to find out what's their next move and I explained to him what had
lead me to the ER. They took my blood pressure which was very
high and took blood test. For the next two hours Destiny, Isaiah
and I just sat and waited for my results. The doc finally came back
and stated "I reviewed your test and everything came back normal
young lady" I believe you had an anxiety attack. "I don't know you
or what you're going through but if I were talking to you as a
friend I would tell you that your stressed and you need to get rid of
it" He gave me a pill which made me a little loopy as Destiny
called it and as I remember correctly he then said "Live life to the
fullest, you have two beautiful children try and cut out the stress as
best you can." He gave me a prescription and sent me on my happy
little anxiety way.

Well that was a wake-up call for me. Try and not stress out.

Easier said than done but I will try and I did but it didn't go the

way I planned.

3 CHAPTER

When we arrived at the hospital we had doctors and nurses running inside and out of the room. Some trying to take vitals of Isaiah, some asking him if he wanted pain medication. It just all was happening so fast and all I could do was stand there and watch. I felt so helpless and I just put my hands over my eyes and began to sob. Why him I just kept saying to myself as my daughter stood beside me and holding me and saying the very same thing but out loud, I wish this was a dream and I could just wake up or even better I wish I were downstairs when it all was beginning and maybe none of this would have happened.

We were at the same hospital in that we were in when he had his first seizure and again it was fully packed with sick people, only this time Isaiah was rushed in on a stretcher and through the back doors straight into a private room. Kevin went with him in the ambulance and I drove my car with my daughter Destiny because she had been screaming and crying while zay was being put on the stretcher and I wasn't fully dressed so I quickly got a pair of jeans on and sweater, some socks and boots and headed off behind the ambulance. Destiny just continued to cry as I drove and kept saying "Mommy zay can't die" and she kept repeating it over and over. I said he's not going to die Des he will be okay and all the while I'm praying to god to keep my son alive and take me instead. He's a good kid he still has a life to live, please god let my son be OK, if you are punishing me I accept it but don't punish him. And as I drifted off in my secret prayer my phone rang. It was my mom. Hello I said, Genelle what happened? Mom I cried, I broke down in tears and Destiny began screaming again. "DESTNY be quiet I can't hear", I understood she was scared but so was I and I know I was supposed to be consoling her but I couldn't while I was driving and trying to watch the rode and hear my mother through the speakerphone of my blackberry. Mommy zay got burned, burned really, I said. Mom help me please. Where are you she asked? We are headed to the hospital and Kevin is with zay in the ambulance. I will meet you there she said and I will call your sister and let her know what happened. Okay I said answered like I was a little girl. It will be alright, zay is a strong little boy you know that, he will get through it she said. Yes, I no. Okay see you soon and Destiny push the end button and we headed to the hospital. As soon as we got to the hospital, we were not too far from the ambulance we parked and ran right in I am Isaiah Edwards mother, where is he? Oh, a nurse said please follow me.

There he was laying on the bed and half his face burned to the bone. All I could do to keep from crying was to hold his hand and try and console him. Soon after my mother and sister Tia arrived and walked in the room and they both just busted down in tears. My sister Tia had to walk out the room and I walked out after her to see how she was and she grabbed me and hugged me like she used to when we were kids. Genelle. She said" I'm so sorry" What happened.? I don't know I told her all I know is while I was upstairs with Destiny, Kevin called me and when I came downstairs he was holding zay in his arms. While I am telling Tia this, I look over and I see a male nurse who was taking care of my son staring and listening to my every word. Not thinking anything of it I continued to tell her everything that happened from there. I called 911 I said and they were asking me questions and I didn't know. I couldn't talk. "Then they asked our address and I began to cry and I couldn't tell them".

Soon after the nurse calls Kevin and I over and ask can he speak with us for a minute, and we did only to find out that we were being reported to the children and youth services by him, (he claimed he had too) but we were foster parents and we knew that he didn't have too, he felt it necessary because we had unanswered questions. We had too much on our minds at the point to really care what that nurse was doing, all we cared about was our son and we wanted to know what happened just like everyone else. I knew that once the case workers heard what was going on they would know that we would never hurt our child on purpose. I'm not going to lie, I was hurt and angry at that nurse. He had no compassion at all, he was all business and had no feelings. But I do understand he had a job to do and if he felt like that was something he had to do, so be it.

We signed the paperwork he asked to signed regarding Isaiah and being hurt and as we walked away all I could was cry. Not because we as parents were being falsely accused of harming my son but because I just felt like everything was crumbling before my very eyes and there was nothing I could do to stop it.

I look back on that day now and I remember feeling so mad at that nurse that I cussed him out something awful in my head and I told Kevin God is watching over him and his spirit and I pray that no one in family gets hurt and treats him the way he treated us. Kevin was so mad that he actually wanted to punch his lights out, but I told him that wouldn't solve a thing but add extra stress to the stress we already have right now. Mind you Kevin can have a temper and I have seen it plenty of times in the fourteen years of marriage. Gratefully he has never gotten arrested and he's never hit the kids or I and I believe in my heart he had it somewhat under control.

After the drama with the nurse I had to go check on Destiny, I no she had to be going through a lot of pain and hurt seeing her little brother like that. I found her in the waiting room with her basketball coach. She played basketball on her high school team and her coaches were very fond of her as a person and as a player. I guess when everything happened she called him and he came right over to the hospital to sit with her for moral support. He brought coffee for Kevin and I and when I walked into the waiting room she had her face covered with her hand balling her eyes out and he was just sitting there and I could hear him saying to her" it will be okay; your brother will overcome this". "If you need me I'm here for you, we are here for you, we as a team or here for you." I walked over just as he was finishing and He stood up to hug me and tell me how sorry he was for all of this. I said thank you and thanked him for being there for Destiny while I was in room with Isaiah. I was grateful for having the support of family, friends, and the coaches. I asked Destiny do you want to see your brother? He's asking for you. She answered in a baby like voice "Mommy no, I can't, I can't see him like that, please don't make me". Right then and there I saw that my daughter was hurting just like I was and I had to be there for both of my children. And I sat with her and hugged her and told it will be alright. Your brother is a strong little man. (we call him a little man with an old soul) If you knew him and talked to him I'm sure would say the same thing. I knew I had to be strong for both of my children as I always had but this time I had to stronger than ever. I wasn't going to let what was happening to distract me from being a mother to my daughter who needed me now more than she had ever needed me before. Destiny was fifteen turning sixteen and although she was big and tall for her age she was a little girl the inside. She and I have always been close and when she needed me I was there. Don't get me wrong as a girl and being a teenager, it wasn't easy. Teenage hormones going, thinking she knew it all, couldn't tell her anything but at the end of the day she was a good kid. We used to go make dates just the two us to go get something to eat and go to the park or go bowling. I loved spending time with her and I was happy that she loved spending time with me.

4 CHAPTER

Isaiah Edwards born in Nyack hospital in upstate New York on September,23, 1998. Three pounds and nine ounces. What a blessing he was to me. He fought for his life in this world and I knew he was and still is destined for greatness. He had more willfulness to and drive to want so much in life. He is what keeps me focused and driven to find help not only for Isaiah but for the three million people in the united states suffering as well.

Isaiah's life was like every other eleven-year-old boy's life. He loved to go outside and skateboard in the driveway and street with his friends. He wanted to be Tony Hawk at one point but only better. He enjoyed playing his video games often. And when he wasn't doing that he wanted to try out karate classes and he became very good too but months after taking it he realized it was something he didn't have passion for he said so I allowed him to quit. He loved to watch wrestling. The wwe and Monday night raw was a regular thing for him. He liked to watch John Cena and Rey

Mysterio. He must have had over a hundred toy wrestling figures, magazines and wrestling rings. And when we could we would take him to a wrestling match in hopes of seeing a famous wrestler and getting an autograph. It never happened but nevertheless he enjoyed the matches. But his true passion was cooking. I remember him as a little boy maybe around five or six asking me could he help with making dinner. I was very surprised but thankful for the offer and would let him help with making the simple things like helping me the biscuits and putting them on the tray or helping me make salad and the homemade dressing to go along with it. Whatever it was I would cook he would always want to help and always stuck behind my back and added his own little flair and touch. I laugh now because he told not too ago that he did that and much better it tasted.

At age eight Isaiah began watching the food network quite often, when other kids were outside riding their bikes and hanging out he would be sitting on the couch watching the chefs on TV and telling me "One day I am going to be a chef and open my own restaurant". I would tell him you can be whatever you want to be and although I know when I would tell people what his plans where they would laugh because what kid his age knows what they want to be at that age. But he knew and he knew recipes of all sought. He always said he wanted to be like his favorite chef Bobby Flay and one day he knew Bobby would come to his restaurant and eat and love his food. I asked him one day "What makes Bobby Flay your favorite from the rest of the chefs on TV? "His simple answer was "He has passion" This kid is wise and has so much wisdom at such a young age.

I remember coming home from school and work one day and I was exhausted and as I pulled into the driveway I could smell the aromas of food cooking but I knew it couldn't come from house. I wasn't home the kids were the only ones there so it left my mind. Once I opened up the door I realized it is my house smelling this good and someone has cooked. There Isaiah was setting the kitchen table making it look all fancy, tablecloth and all. Hi mom he said, hi zay who cooked? "Me but don't worry Destiny turned on the stove and watched me, I know the rules". Just wash your hands and sit down and I will serve you. Listen to this this kid made Smothered chicken with brown gravy, white rice, corn on the cob, salad and biscuits. I was in such awe. He said to me enjoy mommy I know you had a long day and I just wanted to help you. So, I figured I would cook. This became like a regular thing thereafter. He was cooking dinner more and more and getting recipes out of cookbooks I used to read and off the cooking channel he would watch. He even began making up his own recipes as he got more comfortable with seasonings and herbs. He would ask for me to take him to the flea market and fresh fruit market so he could get fresh herbs and vegetables to make his dishes tastes better. This kid was amazing and he loved what he did. He really enjoyed cooking. Later on, as time went on he began to ask for cookbooks as presents or would ask for cooking supplies. Things like Rachael Ray pots or garlic press. This kid knew what he wanted and to be honest when he got these gifts he used them all. He loved to cook and I loved that he loved to cook too especially since that meant I cook put my feet up and watch my mini chef whip up amazing creations.

Among other things of Isaiah's many things of amazing wonders. He loved to be GQ. He took three showers a day and always had to smell nice. (still does by the way). He had a collection of colognes from Usher to Burberry right down to Ralph Lauren Polo. The list could go on for a while so I will just let you imagine. He even had good smelling soaps and body washes. My husband laughs because he would say Isaiah was going to make a good smelling husband one day.

He doesn't cook much anymore like he used to and his dreams of owning a restaurant have changed a little bit. He now wants me to own the restaurant and use his recipes that he calls master recipes. I know it's the fear of cooking and having a seizure since it has happened a couple of times which with the grace of God on our side someone was always there. I understand his fear and for a while I must admit I wouldn't let him cook. But that's not right on my part. He should be able to do what everyone does in the world regardless of what he has. He just has to do it in a different way and I was going to figure it all out. Kevin said I babied Isaiah and

I did. He would say" He's not going to be little forever and then

what will you do?" I knew he was right and I would say in my

mind "Kevin SHUT UP". It's better when someone can't hear you

and you talk junk. Anyway, so I decided to put Isaiah in a cooking

class at the local college Northampton college which is located in

Tannersville PA and is just one of many sites they have. He

attended his first class which was on a Saturday and really enjoyed

it and told me straight upfront "Mom I'm going to beat Bobby Flay

one day" and started laughing. I knew from just that statement

alone my son was coming back to me.

28

5 CHAPTER

Isaiah and I stayed in the hospital for a great length of time. At

one point he was getting so depressed that the doctor suggested to

let him try and go home for a day or two but he would have to keep

his bandages on and they would teach me what I needed too in

order to keep it clean. Yes, there was a lot to remember but I was

like a sponge remembering what I needed and writing down what I

knew I couldn't. I wanted to do whatever it took to make Isaiah

happy again and feel normal and this was it. Friday came and it

was time to be released for the weekend and we were so delighted.

I could tell Isaiah was smiling even though under those tight

bandages covered his whole face I knew that excitement was there.

As the nurse gave me the directions once again and I signed the

release forms we headed home. He was all bandaged up and on his

left side of his face and hand was where the burns occurred so the

nurses came in like clockwork to make sure they put saline on

them both. He began to have a lot of pain so I would make sure that he received his pain medicine every four hours as one of his told me that he could have it for. He was a brave little man, I could tell he would be in pain but he wouldn't complain. He couldn't move his head to much because of all the duoderm he had on him that the nurses from the burn center had placed just the day before he was admitted. I would just sit there and stare at him and wonder what he was thinking and pray that he would be alright. We would have small talks here and there but I could tell that he was angry, but not at me but at everything that happened and the things that were going to happen next.

His surgeon Dr. Ebberman would check in on him every day and give me updates on his progress. This particular day she came in and I almost felt like she had been crying before she entered out room. She was a great surgeon and from I googled about her she was one of the best and I felt blessed to have her taking care of my son. She was a very mild talking woman with blondish hair and had an accent. One I've never heard before and her voice was calming and very reassuring so whenever she came to see Isaiah I was always thrilled. I felt things would be okay with her being his doctor. Besides she's the one who figured out what happened the day of his accident. To me at this point she could do no wrong in my eyes. She was our savior.

I anticipated the worse news but hoped for the best as he sat down beside me and on the bed that I laid in next to Isaiah and told me the devastating news that he was unfortunately burned third degree to the bone and that he would need several surgeries to help him get his skin back. She explained how first they would have to give fake skin on his face and hand and that it would take a week or so adhere and from there they would be able to do a skin graft. I looked over at Isaiah and what he said next warmed my heart but I think Dr. Ebberman got a little choked up. Mommy he said "I trust whatever she is going to do me, I know she will take care of me" I said with a smile on face yes baby, yes, she will. The doctor didn't hear what he said so she asked me what did he say and I began to repeat the words that he just said to me and in that little second, she began to cry. He's a special kid she said. He doesn't know me and to have the trust that he has is an amazing thing. I take care of adults who don't say things like that. I think that very day was the day Dr. Ebberman knew she was going to do everything it took to give my son the best chance of having his face back. She told us in a day two that she would begin putting on the skin and a week later would be doing the skin graft. She explained that the skin they would use would come from his leg and they only needed a small piece and it would be used to cover his face and hand. She also explained how lucky he was because she was going to do everything in her power to fix everything she could. Isaiah had several surgeries. The first one he was given was to put skin on his face first and on his hand as well. It seemed like eternity as Kevin and I waited for his surgery to be done. I must have had five or six coffees that day. I remember I had to go to the bathroom but I didn't want to miss the Dr. coming out giving us little updates. Yes, I know what you're thinking, Kevin is there

6 CHAPTER

The day I dreaded the most had finally come. I had to take the drive from the hospital and go to Isaiah's school and explain to them what happened. On the hour and a half drive there all I could think about was what was I going to say and how would I explain exactly what happened. I couldn't think straight at all. I was already upset because I had to leave my son helpless in the hospital something I didn't do and secondly It hurt me to have to relive that day all over again. So, as I drove to the school I had a conversation in my head as I know we all do, and I must have rehearsed what I would say to them all while not trying to break down and cry.

Well just to let you know my rehearsal in the car didn't work. My eyes began to tear up and it got so bad that I had to pull over on the side of the road and just cry. I guess if you think about it, I needed that cry because I hadn't really let myself do it while in the hospital with Isaiah. I couldn't let him see cry and be down. I had to be there for him in every way. Crying wasn't an option. I guess holding in all in finally took a toll on me and I just belted out a scream. My eyes felt heavy and my body felt numb. I knew I had to get myself together before I arrived at the school so I dried my eyes with some old tissues I had in my coat pocket and pulled my mirror out of my purse and tried my best to look as "Normal" as possible. And I began my journey to the school again.

I made it to the school and as I approached the front door and pushed the security button and looked up at the camera I heard the voice of the woman in the office say "How can I help you" I responded" Yes Hi I am here to talk to the principal about my son Isaiah" And before I could say his last name I was buzzed in. I walked to the security desk to get my visitors pass and sign in the book as everyone had to do when they entered the school and the woman asked me" how is Isaiah doing I haven't seen him lately"?

Now how could this woman ask me this right now I am thinking in my head? But I answered her with "Not good he's in the hospital" and as I told her this I felt that same feeling as I had in the drive to the school and I had to hold my tears back. All I could say was "Thank you for asking, I will tell him you asked about him". I felt bad because I have talked to this woman for numerous years. We spoke several times even when my daughter attended the school years prior to Isaiah attending so I know she knew something was really wrong and I could tell she wanted to know but I just couldn't talk to her at that moment. I had to stay strong and if I talked to her I would break down. "Mrs. Edwards he's ready for you" the receptionist called to me" As I walked in his office I couldn't feel my knees, it felt like I was going to fall over. I felt I was going to have an anxiety attack. I shouldn't have been there by myself. His dad should have come with me and given me support. He wasn't just my son he was his too but as always, I had to do this like I had to do so many other things by myself. And so here I was sitting down in front of the principal letting him know what happened. "Principal… "Good morning How are you" he asked, Me… "Not so good" he looked at me with a puzzled look on his face like he had no idea why I was there. Which I suppose he hadn't. Principal… "Well tell me what is going on? "Me…. Isaiah had a seizure on December 20 and fell onto my wood burning stove and was burned third degree on his face and hand and was burned to the bone, He's in the hospital right now and he's not doing too well" I knew it would come and it did, yep I started crying and he began to tear up as well. He handed me some tissues and I continued to tell him my story. This was his first seizure and we had no idea at the time what happened when he got burned. When we arrived at the hospital they took test and that's when they found out he had a seizure, he has epilepsy. The look on his face I will never forget, I'm used to seeing this man with a smile on his face walking up and down the hallways of the school and Isaiah was very fond of him. All the years that he has been principal he has always treated me with respect, now seeing him at this moment he was silent and it looked like he was getting pale. I know his silence was from listening to me but I couldn't help notice that our conversation seemed to feel personal for some reason and that he was feeling my pain. And he says Principal…." I'm so sorry I know nothing I say can make it any easier on you" "I have kids of my own and I couldn't imagine what you are going through at this time" He came from behind his desk and extended his arms out to me and gave me a hug. A hug I needed. I was glad he listened to me but I felt bad that I had to give him bad news the way I did. Principal… "I am very fond of your son he said" "He's a good boy and student, he's always smiling and gets along with everyone" Please tell him I am thinking of him" Me…." I will thank you so much". Principal…" Do you think he would like cards from his class? "It may bring his spirits up" Me…. "Oh yes thank you, he would love that" "He's been so depressed since he's been in the hospital and he miss school and his friends a lot". Principal… "Give me the name of the hospital and the room number he's staying in and I will send it as soon as possible" Me…" Thank you so much for everything, I really do appreciate it" I won't tell him I will let it be a surprise". Principal…" No don't thank me, it's an honor." And that was it. He gave me a hug again and I left.

On the ride back home, I felt a sense of relief come over me. I knew that I had to talk about it and tell about what happened to Isaiah and I knew it wasn't going to be easy but I did it. And it felt good. I actually Did it! Now I had to put on my brave face and go back to my son. And I headed off.

All while I was driving I was thinking about Isaiah's accident and how I felt it was my fault for not catching his seizure. I remembered when the school nurse called me and let me know she watched him having a seizure in class. I know that I did everything I could but I couldn't still but feel guilty. All sought of questions ran through my mind like what if he was having seizures in front of me and I couldn't tell and I mistake it for him just ignoring me, or my number one question is why I have I never seen one? I had so many questions and no answers and it was just eating away at me all the time.

I finally made it back to the hospital and sat in the car for a few minutes to collect my thoughts and fix my face so Isaiah wouldn't know that I had been crying. I took out my cell phone and called my mother to let her know how my appointment with the principal and told her his class would be sending him get well cards and how happy he will be when they arrived. She was happy and told me I sounded better and that she would be up later to visit and bring me a home cooked meal. I thanked her, told her I loved her and hung up.

I finally made it back to the hospital room and I could tell Isaiah had been waiting for me, as soon as I walked in he said" Finally your back, I missed you" with a smile on his face. "I missed you too bud" and I gave a hug. I sat down on my bed which was a like a couch pushed up against the window and I told him that I talked to his principal and he said to tell him hello and get well soon. He asked did I see any of his teachers and I told him no but I explained what happened to him and the principal would let the teachers know. He then sat up in his bed and had a serious look on his face and said to me" Mom I miss school and all of my friends" I replied" I know you do and you know soon you will be back" "No mom I'm not going back" he said with a loud voice. I could tell he was getting upset by the look in his eyes and the tone in his voice. "Isaiah the doctor said in a couple of months you will be well enough to go back" "No mom I won't, I'm not going back, can't I be home-schooled?" I was in shock I didn't know he didn't want to go back to school. And before I could answer him he laid back down and began to cry and said" Look at me mom, look at my face, I have half of a face mom, I am not going back or anywhere" "But Isaiah" I said "Your surgeries are going so well. Dr. Eberstein is doing such a fabulous job ". He didn't answer me and he actually turned his head the opposite way from me and said" I'm going to take a nap now I don't feel so good" "Okay" I said. I knew now more than ever how important those cards from school would really mean to me and my heart hurt for him. I had no idea he felt the way he did and I was not going to force him to go if he didn't feel comfortable going. He had been through enough as it was.

Later on, my mother came to visit and bought me some of her home cooking. She bought me her famous fried chicken, macaroni and cheese, cornbread and collard greens. It has been awhile since I was able to eat food other than the hospital cafeteria food and was grateful for my mom. She knew I wasn't going to leave her

grandson unless I had too and to leave him to go make myself

some food wasn't at the top of my list. While I ate we talked for a

while about things going on with her and how everyone in her

church were praying for Isaiah. She told him how he was her hero

and told him how strong he was.

7 CHAPTER

In 1998 I married my husband Kevin and I must state that he has been such a support system for me. So many times, I just wanted to give up on myself and he would let me know that giving up wasn't an option. He would always say" Baby if you give up who would take care of the kids the way you do?" "Isaiah needs you, Destiny needs you" It wasn't that I wanted to give up but taking care of Isaiah was tough. I never wanted to go anywhere unless he went with me because I always had that fear that he could have a seizure and I wouldn't be around. I found myself getting depressed because I felt like this man married me intending on going out and having fun and I just couldn't do that. It was tough on me and I'm pretty sure it was tough on him as well but he never complained.

When I first met my husband, he was the love of my life. We did everything together. And what I loved most about him was he was so good with my daughter Destiny who was age three at the time.

He loved her like she was his own child and never once called her stepchild. He came from a family that I call A connected family and he felt like we all were one and that was that. This man loved me and I loved him. And we got married on January, 2, 1998.

I had a schedule that I followed each and every day concerning the kids and exceptionally with Isaiah. I often wondered would he think I was crazy for what I was doing or was I just that dedicated as a mother. My routine was like any other mothers but I was extra careful with Isaiah. By this time Isaiah was going back to school and I knew it wasn't easy for him so I would wake up Monday through Friday at four am and go to work, leave work around seven to get him up dressed and fed so that I could drive him to school. I started doing this because he let me know that he felt very uncomfortable riding on the bus going and coming. Kids can be cruel and some were and some weren't and Isaiah just couldn't deal with it. They would ask him over and over questions concerning to his face like "What happened to your face" or "Does it hurt?"" Can I touch it?" In their defense they were all legitimate questions but he just didn't feel comfortable talking about it. Then there were the mean kids that just wanted to be immensely cruel and call him Freddy from the scary movie or tell nasty jokes about his scars on his face and hand. He felt like an outcast and would come home off the bus filled with rage. I would ask him how his day was and day after day he would cry and tell me what the kids would say and how he hated school and he wasn't going back. I would try and let him know that I understood how he felt and he would scream at the top of his lungs" No Mom you really don't know, you have no idea what I go through" "Why can't you just home school me" As I watched the tears come down his face I knew he was right. I didn't know how he felt, I wasn't in his shoes. Not only did he have to feel different from now having epilepsy but he also had this huge scar on his face and he looked different. It changed him, he was a different Isaiah. He no longer wanted to go out to play, he didn't want to go to school. He was in a shell. And I hurt for him, there was nothing I could do for him. As a parent and mother, you hurt for them when they're in pain and you feel helpless when you can't do anything to fix it for them. So, I made a decision to make him feel as comfortable as much as I could even if that meant I had to drive back and forth to place to place and get up earlier than normal if it meant he would have a decent day.

Some people say that wasn't the smartest move that I did. But to me it was. They didn't have to see my son hurt. I often ask myself now did I make the right decision and I still think I did for this situation.

Chapter 8

Since Isaiah has gotten sick I have been by his side nonstop. Don't get me wrong I know it's my job as his mother and protector but it's not easy. Since his accident and diagnosis of epilepsy I am with him all of the time, I am the person who when he's in a cranky mood gets yelled at, or when he's aggravated, I am the one he lashes out at. Now believe me I know it's not right for him to do. Had it been any other parent they wouldn't have stood for it but at that time when he first got hurt I didn't know what to do. He's my baby and to see him hurting, hurt me. So, I dealt with it. It wasn't easy either I can tell you that. There were plenty days and nights where he was in pain and someone would come in the room to see him and he didn't want to be bothered and he would give me the evil eye as if I was to get rid of them.

I can remember when we were in the hospital and his social worker would come to visit him and he would be so angry, not at her per say but just at what life had just dealt him. He was burned on one side of his face and he now was told he had epilepsy. So, I understand the anger. I would do everything for him, He couldn't do anything for himself at all. He was always in pain and the medications had him drowsy most of the time so good old me wasn't going anywhere. His social worker Ms. Liz would come talk with him and try to get his emotions out and talk with him about everything. Things he liked, things he didn't. His family and school and he just wouldn't respond to her. And I was angry as well, I felt guilty that I was angry. I was angry at myself, my son was burned and I couldn't help him. I was angry at God how could he do this to my son, he is a good kid. So, I guess in my mind I did everything I could possibly do to make him comfortable and try and make him happy again. So, I never left his side. He would yell at me in anger for not fixing his bed right or for his pillow being in the wrong place and I would just do it and say "sorry". Sorry became part of my most words in the vocabulary. I was apologizing almost all day and half the time I didn't know what for but it just became a habit I suppose. I knew this wasn't who he was, he's not that kind of kid so I just dealt with it even though my feelings were hurt and my spirit was even lower. I was his only caretaker although his dad came to the hospital every day, I was the one who bathed him, made his bed, talked to him when he was upset and needed to talk. He needed me and I knew it and nothing or nobody was going to get me away from that room and away from my son. We now had a bond, a bond no one could understand. He needed me to care for him and I needed him to be okay.

One day a woman called my phone and I wasn't up to talking these days but I answered my phone anyway and this woman says "Hi Genelle"" Yes this is she" I answered. Hi my name is Margo and Isaiah's social worker Ms. Lucy asked me to talk to you a little bit if you're up to it. My son also was burned last year and she thought it would be a good idea if we exchanged stories. "Umm no I said. I can't leave Isaiah alone but thanks you" She quickly said I can come to you" Do you drink coffee? I can bring you up a cup and we can chat in the room next store to his room, just for a few minutes. "I hesitated for a minute and in the back of my mind I was mad. Mad as hell. Who is this lady and why is she bothering me? I have everything I need in this room and across the hall. I don't need her coffee and I don't need to talk and then I heard her voice again, You there? "Yes, I am here, sure I will meet you I said but only for a few minutes I can't leave my son for long." Great she said, I will be up around noon" Is that good for you? Sure, I said with anger in my voice I'm sure see you then. All that morning I was wondering how I was going to tell Isaiah that I was meeting some woman I never met and I would be leaving him alone for a while. So, I decided not to until the time would come. He was used to me being in that room with him at all times and never leaving him so I found it difficult to do it even if it was in the next room over. Which I later found out was a family room. A place where anyone could go and relax and get out of their rooms for a while. I didn't feel like relaxing, how could my son be laying in a hospital bed in pain, depressed and half in face burned to the bone, what kind of mother does that I kept thinking.

It was noon and I decided to tell Isaiah that I was meeting with someone his social worker wanted me to meet and that I would be right next door if he needed me. I told him all you have to do is call me and I will be there. "He says okay mom" it's fine go ahead but why are you meeting her anyway? I don't know son, I guess they just want to talk. So, I headed to the family room and there she stood waiting. Genelle she said" Yes Hello I said in an almost silent irritated tone. Hi I'm Marsha and she put her arms out and gave me a hug. How are you she asked" I am good, holding up I answered as I sat down as soon as she released her tight embrace. She began to tell me right away her story about what happened to her son, he too was a burn victim. She began to explain how what I was going through she went through. She told me the story how her son was burned from his neck down and how he was playing with his dad and brother and somehow a fire came into the picture. I don't remember exactly the details now because back then when I was listening to her my mind was elsewhere. All I could think about was Isaiah and what he was doing. I felt guilty leaving him by himself in that room helpless. What if he had to go to the bathroom, I knew all he had to do was push the button for the nurse but I did everything for him he didn't need them. My mind was reckless and I did not want to be there with this woman and she knew it. I sat in that chair with my arms crossed and my legs crossing one another and my body positioned away from her. It wasn't personal against her in any way but I was thinking she could have talked to me in Isaiah's room. In my head I'm saying lady leave me alone I know what you're trying to do and it's not working. Go away, just go away. I was feeling overwhelmed, overwhelmed to the point that I think I was getting depressed. I've never experienced depression but from what I was told about it, it felt like I had it. But she hadn't gone away so after ten minutes of spending sharing her story time I decided to just be there in the moment and get it over with so I could hurry up and get back.

After she shared her story I learned many things. One thing was being that I was not alone in this. I wasn't the only mother whose child ever got burned or hurt for that matter and I also figured out that talking helps. I'm not one who normally can express my feelings to people much like talk about my personal issues. I've always been that way and its hurt plenty of my relationships. I've always wanted people see how strong and independent I was, that I didn't need anyone or anything. Even though I knew that was true nor the case, I had did it for so long that it just became natural to me. There was only one person in my life that knew me so well that would put me on blast as we say in slang and that was my god-sister Miriam. She knew everything about me from the good to the bad, from the happy to the sad. We were open with one another about everything and our trust in one another was like no other. She knew how I was feeling and she didn't judge me. Not that anyone did not to my knowledge but it was just easier to vent my frustration, my hurt, my fears and my emotions to her. We both have did that to one another for years without judgment and I guess that's why we remained so close for over thirty years. She wasn't just my god sister but she was my best friend. She knew how to calm me down when no one else could. I remember when I first called her and told her about Isaiah's accident. Before I even could get the whole sentence, she could hear it in my voice something was wrong and screamed "What happened G"? You okay? No zay got burned, wait what? Zay got burned I said" How oh my god" wait. As I'm trying to tell her my voice starts to quiver and my heart feels like it's going to jump out of my chest and I say softly Isaiah had an accident and he fell on the wood burning stove and burned his face third degree. G are you serious she said and I can remember her just crying and yelling what happened I don't understand. I explained to her that they said that he had a seizure and he fell into the stove and how Kevin found him and the whole ordeal with the two hospitals. As I am telling her I could tell that after the initial shock of it all she wished she was there with me. And I knew if she were she would be hugging me and talking to me and doing everything she could do to take some of the pressure

off of me. So how is zay? He's good considering. He's more

concerned with if I'm okay then himself. He's suffering but this is

an excellent burn care hospital and I have faith that he will heal

and everything will go back to normal. I said that but in my heart, I

was praying that it would become true.

9 CHAPTER

It's very difficult seeing your children go through things that are out of your control

and we as parents know this but that don't make it any easier on us. Now that Isaiah is

a teenager he wants his independence, his freedom as he calls it. I now had to come

with the terms that my baby is growing up and I can't be there for him all of the time.

 And with that said" I'm hurt". My daughter Destiny told me that he talks to her

sometimes and explained that I needed to back off from him some and that I could be

 very annoying to him. I had no knowledge that my checking up on him every hour in the middle of the night with the absolute silence was upsetting him. He never shared

that with me. I only did this because he has seizures in his sleep. And months prior to

me doing my nightly check-ups as I call them I did some research on the internet and

found out about something called Sudden unexpected death in epilepsy also known as

 SUDEP. This is a term used when a person has epilepsy suddenly dies, and the reason

for the death is unexplained. As I look into it more I found that approximately 50,000

people die each year in the USA SUDEP. About 1 in 100 sufferers of severe epilepsy die

every year. So, with this information how I could I not check up on my son.

Destiny told me how he was very upset with me and just couldn't understand how

obsessed I have become with epilepsy and him. As she continued telling me his

frustrations with me I began to cry. "Destiny you know I don't mean it" "I'm just doing

what mothers do which is love their children" "I know mom she said but you go too far

sometimes, you do it with the both of us".

I guess from now on I will have to be more creative in sneaking up on him and checking on him.

Final Thoughts

Isaiah wanted me to write this book so that we could bring some type of awareness to epilepsy. He wanted to tell his story of what happened to him as well to tell people to never take life for granted. He was a healthy and happy baby, and one day this just happened with no known cause.

We tend to take things for granted we take people for granted without even realizing it. We get upset with people and stop talking to them. It's not worth it. Life is to precious. We need to live our lives to the fullest because life is not promised to you tomorrow.

Isaiah is living life happy now, he's finding that he enjoys doing different things then he did before. He's loving life and I love him

Author's Bio

Genelle Manso is a mother to Destiny and Isaiah and grandmother to Damian.

Genelle resides in the Pocono's Pa with her two children and grandson. She is an author

and currently in college to get her bachelor's degree in nursing. Genelle also is the CEO of her

charity she started as well as a Facebook group called Epilepsy Angels.